THE USE OF

APPLE CIDER VINEGAR

WEIGHT LOSS RESOLUTION RECIPE

TRANSFORMATIVE HEALTH BENEFIT OF USING ACV DIET NATURALLY TO SHED POUNDS, GUT HEALTH CARE, SKIN CONDITIONS ETC

KATE CASTILLO

Table of Contents

Introduction to Apple Cider Vinegar

Apple cider vinegar (ACV), made from fermented apple cider, has been used for centuries in various cultures for its medicinal properties and culinary versatility. In this comprehensive introduction, we will delve into the origins of ACV, its production process, nutritional composition, and a variety of purported health benefits.

- Origins and History

The use of vinegar as a medicinal and culinary agent can be traced back thousands of years to ancient civilizations like the Babylonians, Egyptians, Greeks, and Romans, who all valued its potential health benefits and food preservation properties. Evidence suggests that vinegar was discovered by accident around 5000 BC, when unattended grape juice turned into wine and then into vinegar.

Historically, apple cider vinegar was used not only in cooking, but also as a natural remedy for ailments ranging from digestive issues to skin conditions. Apples, a fruit widely cultivated across Europe and Asia, provided an ideal base for creating a vinegar with a distinct fruity flavor profile.

- Production Process

The fermentation of apple cider is the first step in making apple cider vinegar. This process consists of many important steps:

Apple Selection: High-quality apples are picked, usually a mix of sweet and tart kinds to provide a balanced flavor profile.

Pressing involves crushing the apples to extract the juice, which is then filtered to eliminate any solid particles.

Fermentation begins with the addition of yeast to apple juice, which converts the sugars into alcohol and produces apple cider.

Acetic Acid Fermentation: To convert apple cider into vinegar, acetic acid bacteria (acetobacter) are added to the cider, which converts the alcohol into acetic acid via a secondary fermentation process.

Maturation: Vinegar is aged in tanks or barrels for several weeks to months to create its distinct flavor and acidity.

Filtration and bottling: Once matured, the vinegar is filtered to eliminate sediment before being bottled for distribution.

The conventional method of making apple cider vinegar incorporates natural fermentation processes that retain its nutritional value and therapeutic components.

- Nutritional Composition

Apple cider vinegar is loved not just for its tart flavor, but also for its nutritional content. While particular nutritional values can vary slightly depending on the brand and manufacturing processes, normal apple cider vinegar provides the following nutrients per tablespoon (15 ml):

Approximately 3 calories:

Carbohydrates: Negligible amount, usually less than 1 gram.

- Acetic acid is the principal active ingredient in vinegar, accounting for approximately 5-6% of its content.
- Other acids include citric, malic, and lactic acids.

Potassium: little levels, perhaps 11 mg.

- Although low in vital nutrients, apple cider vinegar is known for its bioactive components, particularly acetic acid, which is thought to contribute to many of its health advantages.

- Health Benefits of Apple Cider Vinegar

While anecdotal evidence and preliminary studies support many of the alleged health benefits of apple cider vinegar, more rigorous clinical research is required to fully establish the extent of ACV's therapeutic potential. The following are some of the key potential benefits:

Digestive Health: ACV may help digestion by increasing stomach acid production and encouraging the growth of good gut flora.

Blood Sugar Regulation: According to some research, ACV can enhance insulin sensitivity and lower blood sugar levels after meals, which may assist people who are insulin resistant or have type 2 diabetes.

Weight Management: ACV may help reduce hunger and increase feelings of fullness, resulting in lower calorie consumption and possible weight loss over time.

Heart Health: Preliminary study suggests that ACV may help lower cholesterol and blood pressure, lowering the risk of heart disease.

antibacterial qualities: Acetic acid, the primary component of ACV, has antibacterial qualities that may help suppress the growth of pathogens such as bacteria and fungi.

Skin and Hair Care: Diluted ACV can be applied topically to promote skin health, balance pH levels, and increase hair shine.

- Practical applications

Incorporating apple cider vinegar into your daily routine may be simple and pleasurable. Here are some useful suggestions and ideas for using ACV:

To make a tangy salad dressing, combine ACV, olive oil, mustard, honey, and herbs.

In Beverages: For a pleasant morning tonic, combine a tablespoon of ACV, water, lemon juice, and honey.

Cooking: Use ACV to enhance the flavor of sauces, marinades, and soups.

Diluted ACV can be used as a natural household cleanser because of its antibacterial characteristics.

Apple cider vinegar (ACV) is more than just a condiment; it is a versatile and potentially beneficial addition to your health and wellness regimen. While its traditional uses and anecdotal benefits have been known for centuries, ongoing research continues to uncover new insights into its therapeutic properties. Whether you want to support digestion, manage blood sugar levels, or enhance the flavor of your favorite dishes, ACV provides a natural and accessible solution.

As you explore the world of apple cider vinegar, remember to choose high-quality, organic varieties to ensure maximum nutritional benefits. Incorporate ACV into your daily routine in moderation, and consult with a healthcare professional if you have specific health concerns or conditions. Accept the tangy goodness of apple cider vinegar and discover how it can contribute to your overall well-being.

Chapter 1

Health Benefits of Apple Cider Vinegar

Apple cider vinegar (ACV), derived from fermented apple cider, has gained popularity in recent years for its potential health benefits, which are supported by both traditional wisdom and emerging scientific research. In this comprehensive exploration, we will delve into the various health benefits attributed to apple cider vinegar, examining the scientific evidence behind them.

- Digestive Health

One of the most well-known benefits of apple cider vinegar is its potential to support digestive health. ACV is believed to aid digestion primarily by increasing stomach acid production, which is necessary for efficient food breakdown and nutrient absorption. Many people who experience digestive discomfort, such as bloating or indigestion, report relief after consuming diluted apple cider vinegar.

Mechanism & Evidence

Acetic acid, the main active component of ACV, is thought to stimulate the secretion of digestive enzymes and increase the acidity of the stomach. This acidic environment is conducive to the breakdown of proteins into amino acids and the activation of digestive enzymes like pepsin, which further aids digestion.

While there is anecdotal evidence supporting ACV's digestive benefits, scientific studies have produced mixed results. Some animal studies suggest that acetic acid may improve gastric emptying rate and decrease the time food stays in the stomach, potentially alleviating symptoms of indigestion and reflux. However, more human studies are needed to confirm these effects conclusively.

- Practical Application

To improve digestive health, try incorporating apple cider vinegar into your daily routine in the following ways:

Dilute 1-2 tablespoons of ACV in a glass of water and drink 15-30 minutes before meals to improve digestion.

As a Salad Dressing: Use ACV as the base for homemade salad dressings to aid digestion while enjoying a healthy dinner.

After Meals: Consuming diluted ACV after meals can help relieve bloating and discomfort.

- Blood Sugar Regulation

Another interesting aspect of apple cider vinegar is its ability to assist manage blood sugar levels, especially after high-carbohydrate meals. This advantage is especially important for people who have insulin resistance or type 2 diabetes.

Mechanism & Evidence

Several small-scale studies have suggested that consuming apple cider vinegar with meals may improve insulin sensitivity and lower blood glucose levels. The acetic acid in ACV is thought to inhibit the digestion of complex carbohydrates, slowing the rate at which sugar enters the bloodstream after eating. This can help prevent blood sugar spikes and reduce the insulin response required to manage those spikes.

A study published in the Journal of Functional Foods discovered that consuming apple cider vinegar before a high-carbohydrate meal significantly reduced blood glucose levels in healthy adults; however, more extensive and long-term studies are needed to fully understand the potential of ACV as an adjunct therapy for diabetes management.

- Practical Application

If you are interested in regulating blood sugar levels using ACV, consider the following practical tips:

Before Meals: Dilute 1-2 teaspoons of ACV in water and drink before meals to potentially reduce the effect of carbs on blood sugar levels.

In beverages, combine ACV with herbal teas or lemon water to create a delicious drink that promotes blood sugar balance.

Consistency: Regular, moderate ACV consumption may produce longer-term advantages for blood sugar management.

- Weight Management

Apple cider vinegar (ACV) has grown in popularity among those looking for natural weight reduction aids. While it is not a cure-all, ACV may help through a variety of processes.

Mechanism & Evidence
Some studies suggest that acetic acid can increase feelings of fullness and reduce the overall amount of food consumed during a meal, which may lead to lower calorie intake over time and potentially support weight loss efforts.

Furthermore, ACV's impact on blood sugar levels and insulin sensitivity may indirectly contribute to weight control. By stabilizing blood sugar levels and lowering insulin spikes, ACV may help avoid cravings and subsequent consumption of high calorie foods.

However, it is important to remember that the evidence for ACV's role in weight control is preliminary; while some studies have showed encouraging outcomes in animals and short human trials, further study is needed to determine its long-term usefulness and safety.

Practical Application
Consider the following practical ideas for incorporating ACV into your weight control routine:

Before meals, drink a glass of water with 1-2 teaspoons of apple cider vinegar to potentially reduce hunger and calorie consumption.

In Recipes: Mix ACV into marinades, sauces, and salad dressings to add taste and maybe increase satiety.

Healthy Lifestyle: When attempting to lose weight, ACV should be considered as part of a balanced diet and regular physical activity.

- Heart Health

New research reveals that apple cider vinegar may have heart-health benefits, particularly in terms of decreasing cholesterol and improving blood pressure.

Mechanism & Evidence

Acetic acid, the active component in ACV, has been studied for its potential effects on lipid metabolism. Animal studies have shown that acetic acid can reduce total cholesterol, triglycerides, and LDL (bad) cholesterol levels while increasing HDL (good) cholesterol levels. These effects are thought to be due to ACV's ability to enhance the expression of genes involved in lipid metabolism.

In terms of blood pressure, some animal studies suggest that acetic acid may help lower blood pressure by inhibiting the activity of the enzyme renin, which regulates blood pressure. Although human studies are limited, preliminary evidence suggests that regular consumption of apple cider vinegar may support cardiovascular health via these mechanisms.

- Practical Application

To boost heart health with ACV, consider the following practical applications:

Incorporate ACV into your daily diet: Cooking and meal preparation might help you benefit from its advantages on cholesterol and blood pressure.

Consistent drinking: Regular, moderate drinking of ACV may be essential for preserving possible cardiovascular benefits over time.

Consultation: If you have any current cardiac diseases or concerns, consult with your doctor before introducing ACV into your daily regimen.

- Antimicrobial properties

Apple cider vinegar's acetic acid component is principally responsible for its antibacterial capabilities, which have been recognized in traditional medicine for ages.

Mechanism & Evidence

Acetic acid (ACV) generates an acidic environment that prevents the growth of germs and fungi, making it a popular choice for natural cleaning solutions, food preservation, and even mild skin ailments.

Acetic acid has been demonstrated in studies to successfully prevent the growth of pathogens including E. coli and Candida albicans. This antimicrobial activity applies to both internal and external uses of ACV, making it a versatile alternative for maintaining hygiene and supporting general health.

- Practical Application

Consider the following practical applications for ACV's antibacterial properties:

Cleaning Solution: Make a natural household cleanser by diluting ACV with water and applying it to surfaces.

Food Preservation: Use ACV as a pickling agent to preserve vegetables and extend their shelf life.

Topical Application: Apply diluted ACV to the skin to treat small cuts, bug bites, and fungal infections (always conduct a patch test first and dilute adequately).

- Skin and Hair Care

Aside from its internal health benefits, apple cider vinegar is regarded for its potential use in skincare and hair care.

Mechanism & Evidence

When applied topically, diluted apple cider vinegar can help:

Skin: Restore pH balance, treat acne, soothe sunburn, and enhance overall skin texture.

Hair: Increase shine, reduce product buildup, and clarify the scalp.

While individual results vary, many people report better skin and hair health after including diluted ACV into their beauty routines.

- Practical Application

To integrate ACV into your skincare and hair care routine, consider these practical tips:

Facial Toner: Combine equal amounts ACV and water, apply to the face with a cotton pad, and rinse after a few minutes for balanced skin.

Hair Rinse: After shampooing, dilute ACV with water (1:1) and apply to hair as a last rinse to remove buildup and add shine.

Caution: Dilute ACV thoroughly before putting it to the skin or hair to avoid irritation or bad reactions.

- Safety Concerns and Precautions

While apple cider vinegar has potential health advantages, it must be used cautiously and with awareness of the hazards.

ACV is highly acidic, and undiluted ingestion can cause discomfort or damage to tooth enamel, throat, or digestive tract. Always dilute ACV with water or other liquids before usage.

Interaction with Medications: If you take insulin or diuretics on a regular basis, see your doctor first because ACV may interact with some medications.

Allergic Reactions: Some people may be allergic to apples or develop allergic reactions to ACV; if you have any side effects, discontinue consumption and consult a doctor.

Apple cider vinegar (ACV) continues to pique the interest of researchers and health enthusiasts alike due to its potential health benefits and diverse applications, which range from supporting digestive health and blood sugar regulation to potentially aiding weight loss and promoting heart health.

As with any natural remedy, it's important to approach ACV with caution and awareness of personal health needs. Gradually incorporate ACV into your diet and skincare routine, observe how your body reacts, and consult with a healthcare provider if you have specific health concerns or conditions.

Accept the traditional wisdom and scientific studies surrounding apple cider vinegar, and learn how this simple yet effective vinegar can help you achieve optimal health and wellness.

Chapter 2

Incorporating ACV into Your Daily Routine

In this comprehensive guide, we'll explore various practical ways to incorporate apple cider vinegar (ACV) into your daily life. ACV has gained popularity not only as a culinary ingredient, but also as a versatile health tonic with a range of potential benefits. Whether you're looking to support digestion, manage blood sugar levels, promote weight loss, or improve skin and hair health, incorporating ACV into your daily routine can be both simple and enjoyable.

- Understanding ACV Types and Quality.

Before we get into how to use ACV, it's important to understand the many types and quality available:

Raw, unfiltered ACV retains the "mother," a murky substance composed of helpful enzymes, proteins, and bacteria. The mother is responsible for many of ACV's health benefits.

Filtered ACV has been treated to remove the mother and sediment, and while it may still provide some advantages, it lacks the entire range of nutrients found in raw, unfiltered forms.

Organic ACV is created using organically cultivated apples, which are free of synthetic pesticides and fertilizers. Choosing organic assures that you consume a product with minimal chemical residues.

Pasteurized ACV is heated to destroy germs and lengthen its shelf life, but unpasteurized ACV maintains more nutrients and beneficial bacteria but must be refrigerated to avoid deterioration.

To enhance potential health advantages, use raw, unfiltered, and organic ACV.

- Practical Tips for Using ACV

Now let's look at some practical and innovative methods to include ACV into your everyday routine:

1. Morning Routine.

Begin your day on a healthy note by incorporating ACV into your morning routine.

ACV Detox Drink: Combine 1-2 teaspoons of ACV with warm water, a squeeze of lemon juice, and a touch of honey or maple syrup. This mixture can help alkalize your body, assist digestion, and increase hydration.

Smoothies: To add a tangy touch to your morning smoothie, mix in a splash of ACV with fruits like apples, berries, or citrus.

2. Salad dressings and sauces.

ACV is a great base for homemade dressings and sauces.

Basic Vinaigrette: For a basic salad dressing, combine ACV, olive oil, Dijon mustard, garlic, salt, and pepper; adjust the ratios to your liking.

ACV's acidity helps tenderize proteins while giving a delicate sour flavor, making it ideal for marinating meats, tofu, or vegetables.

3. Cooking and baking.
Extend your culinary repertoire with ACV-infused dishes:

Soups and stews: To lighten flavors and balance richness and depth, add a splash of ACV near the end of cooking.

ACV, when coupled with baking soda, causes a chemical reaction that allows baked items to rise without the use of eggs or yeast.

4. Beverages
ACV can be put into a variety of beverages to enhance flavor and health benefits.

Herbal Teas: Combine ACV with herbal teas like chamomile or ginger to create a calming beverage that accentuates the herbal flavors while potentially aiding digestion.

Mocktails: Mix ACV with sparkling water, fruit juices, and fresh herbs to make a delightful mocktail. Garnish with lemon slices for a fizzy and flavorful drink.

5. Skincare and Hair Care

Incorporate ACV into your skincare and haircare routines to reap additional benefits.

Facial Toner: To balance pH levels, tighten pores, and minimize acne, dilute ACV with water (1:1 ratio) and apply to clean face with a cotton pad.

After shampooing, rinse your hair with a 1:1 mixture of ACV and water to remove buildup, restore luster, and clarify the scalp, then thoroughly rinse with water.

- Specific Applications of ACV for Health Benefits

1. Digestive Health.

ACV can improve digestive health in a variety of ways:

Before meals, drink a glass of water with 1-2 tablespoons of apple cider vinegar to stimulate digestive enzymes and support healthy digestion.

Incorporate into Recipes: Add ACV to marinades, salad dressings, and sauces to improve flavor and digestion with each meal.

2. Blood Sugar Regulation

To potentially assist control blood sugar levels:

Pre-Meal Consumption: To reduce the influence of carbs on blood sugar levels, take ACV before meals. Dilute it in water or mix it into beverages like tea.

Regular, moderate consumption of ACV may help with long-term blood sugar management, but see your doctor if you have diabetes or insulin resistance.

3. Weight Management.
ACV may help with weight management efforts.

Appetite Control: Drink ACV-infused beverages before meals to increase feelings of fullness and perhaps lower calorie consumption.

Incorporate into Cooking: Use ACV to add taste to foods without adding calories, making them more satisfying.

4. Heart Health.
ACV may have the following potential heart health benefits:

Incorporate ACV into your diet by using it in recipes and dressings as part of a heart-healthy diet; its possible effects on cholesterol and blood pressure may help with cardiovascular health.

Moderation and Balance: To promote heart health, include ACV as part of a well-balanced diet and frequent exercise.

- Safety Concerns and Precautions

While ACV has potential health benefits, it's important to utilize it wisely.

To avoid discomfort or injury to the teeth, throat, or digestive tract, always dilute ACV before consumption. Begin with lesser amounts and modify as needed.

Interaction with Medications: If you take insulin or diuretics on a regular basis, see your doctor first because ACV may interact with some medications.

Allergic Reactions: Some people may be allergic to apples or develop allergic reactions to ACV; if you have any side effects, discontinue consumption and consult a doctor.

- Incorporating ACV into various lifestyles

Whether you have a specific diet or lifestyle, ACV may be tailored to your preferences and needs.

Vegan and vegetarian diets: Add ACV to plant-based foods for a tart flavor and probable digestive benefits.

Paleo & Keto Diets: ACV is naturally low in carbs and can be used sparingly to impart acidity to foods without drastically altering macronutrient ratios.

Gluten-Free and Dairy-Free Diets: Because ACV is naturally gluten-free and dairy-free, it is an adaptable component for individuals following dietary restrictions.

Incorporating apple cider vinegar into your daily routine can enhance your overall well-being through its potential health benefits and culinary versatility. Whether you're looking to support digestion, regulate blood sugar levels, lose weight, or improve skin and hair health, ACV provides a natural and accessible solution.

To harness the power of this ancient remedy in modern life, choose high-quality, organic ACV and experiment with a variety of applications, from morning detox drinks to flavorful salad dressings and beyond. Remember to start slowly, observe how your body responds, and consult with a healthcare provider if you have specific health concerns or conditions.

Embrace the tangy goodness of apple cider vinegar and discover how it may complement your journey toward optimal health and wellness. With creativity and mindfulness, including ACV into your daily routine can be both a health-conscious choice and a flavorful addition to your life.

Chapter 3

Simple ACV Detox Drinks: Maximizing the Health Benefits of Apple Cider Vinegar

Apple cider vinegar (ACV) has gained a reputation as a powerful health tonic, celebrated for its potential detoxifying effects and numerous health benefits. Incorporating ACV into detox drinks is a popular way to enjoy its cleansing properties while enhancing hydration and supporting overall well-being. In this detailed exploration, we'll delve into the science behind ACV detox drinks, explore various recipes tailored to different health goals, and provide practical tips for

- Understanding Detoxification and ACV

Detoxification is the process of eliminating toxins and harmful substances from the body. While our organs, such as the liver and kidneys, naturally perform detoxification, certain foods and beverages can support these processes. ACV is thought to aid detoxification primarily because of its high acetic acid content and possible antioxidant properties.

- Mechanism & Evidence

ACV is mostly made up of acetic acid, which has been researched for its ability to stimulate detoxification pathways in the liver. The liver is responsible for detoxifying toxic compounds and metabolizing lipids, proteins, and carbs.

ACV includes antioxidants, including as polyphenols, which can help neutralize free radicals and reduce oxidative stress in the body. This antioxidant activity may improve general cellular health and detoxification processes.

While scientific research on ACV's particular detoxification effects in humans is lacking, anecdotal data and preliminary studies indicate that integrating ACV into a well-balanced diet may assist promote natural detoxification pathways and general health.

- Benefits of ACV Detox Drinks

ACV detox drinks are a handy and delightful way to get the possible health advantages of apple cider vinegar, which include:

Hydration: Detox beverages produced with ACV frequently include water or other hydrating liquids, which aids in maintaining correct hydration levels, which are critical for general health and wellness.

Digestive Support: ACV may promote digestion by increasing stomach acid production and gut health, which can help with overall detoxification efforts.

Metabolism Boost: According to some studies, ACV may help boost metabolism, perhaps aiding weight loss objectives when combined with a healthy diet and exercise.

Antioxidant Support: The antioxidants in ACV may help resist oxidative stress and free radical damage, thereby promoting cellular health and detoxification processes.

- Practical Guidelines for Making ACV Detox Drinks

ACV detox drinks are simple to make and may be modified to individual preferences and health goals. Here are some helpful hints for preparing and drinking them:

1. The Basic ACV Detox Drink Recipe

This basic recipe can be modified with additional ingredients to suit your preferences:

Ingredients:

- Combine 1-2 tablespoons of raw, unfiltered ACV with the mother.
- 8-12 ounces of water (room or warm)
- Optional: 1-2 teaspoons honey or maple syrup (for sweetness).

Instructions:

- Combine the ACV and water in a glass.
- If desired, mix in honey or maple syrup until thoroughly incorporated.
- Enjoy right away, especially before meals or in the morning as part of a daily routine.

2. Variations of ACV Detox Drink

ACV detox drinks can be customized by adding ingredients that enhance their flavor and potential health benefits.

Citrus Twist: To add a delicious citrus flavor and more vitamin C to your ACV detox drink, pour in some fresh lemon or lime juice.

Herbal Infusions: Steep herbal teas like chamomile, mint, or ginger in hot water, then add ACV and honey for a calming and aromatic detox beverage.

Spiced Elixir: Add warming spices like cinnamon, turmeric, or cayenne pepper to your ACV detox drink for more flavor and possibly metabolic benefits.

Green Tea Boost: Brew green tea and let it cool before adding ACV and a splash of honey. Green tea is high in antioxidants and may help with ACV's detoxification properties.

3. Timing and frequency.
To optimize the potential advantages of ACV detox drinks, consider the following timing and frequency guidelines:

Morning Ritual: Drink an ACV detox drink on an empty stomach or before breakfast to boost your metabolism and encourage hydration after sleep.

Pre-Meal: Drink an ACV detox drink 15-30 minutes before your meal to potentially aid digestion and lower the glycemic reaction to carbohydrates.

Incorporate ACV detox drinks into your daily routine for continuous hydration and possible health advantages. Begin with a lesser dose of ACV and gradually increase as tolerated.

Tailoring ACV Detox Drinks for Specific Health Goals

ACV detox drinks can be customized to meet specific health objectives and preferences. Here are some recipes to help with various elements of health and well-being:

1. Digestive Support Detox Drink.

Ingredients:

- 1–2 teaspoons of raw, unfiltered ACV
- Eight ounces of warm water.
- 1 teaspoon freshly grated ginger (or ginger powder).
- Optional: one teaspoon of honey.

Instructions:

- Combine ACV, warm water, and grated ginger in a mug.
- Stir thoroughly until all ingredients are incorporated.
- If you want it sweeter, add some honey.
- Sip carefully and enjoy the calming benefits of digestion.

2. Metabolism-Boosting Detox Drink.

Ingredients:

- 1–2 teaspoons of raw, unfiltered ACV
- Eight to twelve ounces of cold water
- Juice from 1/2 a lemon
- A pinch of cayenne pepper (optional).
- Optional: Stevia or honey for sweetness.

Instructions:

- In a glass, combine apple cider vinegar, cold water, lemon juice, and cayenne pepper.
- Mix thoroughly until all items are integrated.
- If desired, add stevia or honey to adjust the sweetness.
- Enjoy chilled for a pleasant, metabolism-boosting beverage.

3. An antioxidant-rich detox drink

Ingredients:

- 1–2 teaspoons of raw, unfiltered ACV
- 8 ounces of brewed green tea, chilled
- 1 teaspoon raw honey.
- Optional: Fresh mint leaves for garnish.

Instructions:

- Brew green tea and allow it to cool to room temperature.
- In a glass, blend cooled green tea, ACV, and honey.
- Stir thoroughly until the honey has dissolved.
- Garnish with fresh mint leaves if preferred.
- Enjoy this delicious and antioxidant-rich cleansing beverage.

Additional Tips for Including ACV Detox Drinks

1. Quality Matters

To maximize the potential health benefits, choose high-quality, organic ACV with the mother, which should be raw, unfiltered, and free of preservatives and artificial substances.

2. Gradual introduction.
If you're new to ACV detox drinks, start with lower concentrations and gradually increase as your body adjusts. Monitor how you feel after ingesting ACV to identify the best dosage and frequency for you.

3. Stay hydrated.
Incorporate ACV detox beverages as part of a balanced hydration program; drink plenty of water throughout the day to maintain overall hydration and increase ACV's detoxifying benefits.

4. Consultation with the healthcare provider.
Before introducing ACV detox drinks into your regimen, speak with a healthcare provider if you have any special health problems or diseases, as they can provide personalized advice based on your personal health state and medications.

Safety considerations
While ACV detox drinks are typically healthy for most individuals to use in moderation, it's important to exercise caution:

Dilution: Always dilute ACV with water or other liquids to avoid irritation of the throat, stomach, or tooth enamel.

Interaction with Medications: If you take insulin or diuretics on a regular basis, see your doctor first because ACV may interact with some medications.

Allergic Reactions: Some people may be allergic to apples or develop allergic reactions to ACV; if you have any side effects, stop using it and consult your doctor.

By experimenting with different recipes and incorporating ACV into your daily routine, you can discover a refreshing and health-promoting addition to your lifestyle. ACV detox drinks provide a convenient and flavorful way to harness the potential health benefits of apple cider vinegar, which range from supporting digestion and metabolism to promoting overall detoxification and hydration.

Start gradually, listen to your body's response, and enjoy the tangy goodness of ACV as part of your journey toward optimal health and wellness. Whether you want to boost your metabolism in the morning, soothe digestion with a ginger-infused tonic, or indulge in an antioxidant-rich green tea elixir, ACV detox drinks can be tailored to your preferences and health goals.

Chapter 4

ACV salad dressings and sauces: enhancing flavor and providing health benefits

Apple cider vinegar (ACV) is a versatile ingredient that can transform ordinary salads and dishes into flavorful culinary experiences while potentially offering health benefits. Its tangy flavor and acidity make it an ideal base for salad dressings and sauces, enhancing not only taste but also potentially providing digestive support and other health-promoting properties. In this comprehensive guide, we'll explore the science behind ACV's be

Understanding the role of ACV in salad dressings and sauces
ACV is made from fermented apple cider and contains acetic acid, which gives it its characteristic sour taste and potent health benefits. When used in salad dressings and sauces, ACV not only adds depth and tang but also serves as a natural preservative and flavor enhancer.

- Mechanism and Health Benefits

ACV is high in acetic acid, which has antibacterial effects and may aid digestion by increasing stomach acid production. It also helps balance flavors in dressings and sauces.

Gut Health Support: When ACV is fermented, it generates beneficial bacteria and enzymes known as the "mother," which can help with gut health and digestion.

ACV includes antioxidants, such as polyphenols, which can help neutralize free radicals and reduce oxidative stress in the body, thereby improving overall health and well-being.

Health Advantages of Including ACV in Salad Dressings and Sauces

Adding ACV to salad dressings and sauces can provide a variety of potential health benefits:

Digestive Support: The acetic acid in ACV may increase the synthesis of digestive enzymes, aiding in food breakdown and potentially improving digestion.

Blood Sugar Regulation: According to some studies, ACV may help lower blood sugar levels after high-carbohydrate meals, making it a useful supplement for people managing their blood sugar.

Weight Management: When combined with a balanced diet, ACV's ability to increase feelings of satiety and reduce overall calorie intake may help with weight loss efforts.

Antimicrobial Properties: The acidity of ACV can limit the growth of dangerous germs, potentially aiding in food preservation and safety.

Practical Instructions for Making ACV Salad Dressings

Creating tasty and healthful salad dressings using ACV is simple and allows for unlimited variants to suit varied tastes and preferences. Here are some useful tips:

1. The Basic ACV Salad Dressing Recipe

This core recipe can be used to make a number of ACV salad dressings.

Ingredients:

- 1/4 cup of raw, unfiltered ACV
- 1/2 cup extra virgin olive oil.
- 1 tablespoon Dijon mustard.
- 1 clove minced garlic (optional)
- Add salt and pepper to taste.

Instructions:

- In a small bowl or jar, blend the ACV, olive oil, Dijon mustard, minced garlic (if using), salt, and pepper until well combined.
- Season to taste.
- Use immediately or refrigerate in a tight container for up to a week.

2. Variations on ACV Salad Dressing

ACV salad dressings can be customized with additional ingredients to boost flavor and nutritional benefits.

Honey Mustard Vinaigrette: To make a sweet and tangy dressing, combine 1 tablespoon honey with 1 tablespoon whole grain mustard in the original recipe.

Creamy Balsamic: For a creamy texture, replace some of the ACV with balsamic vinegar and stir in 2 tablespoons of Greek yogurt or mayonnaise.

Citrus Herb Dressing: For a delightful citrus twist, replace some of the ACV with freshly squeezed lemon or orange juice, then add chopped herbs such as parsley, dill, or basil.

3. How to Use ACV in Sauces
ACV can also be added to sauces for cooked dishes to provide acidity and depth of flavor.

Barbecue Sauce: Mix ACV, tomato paste, honey, Worcestershire sauce, and spices to make a tangy barbecue sauce that goes well with grilled meats and veggies.

To add flavor and tenderness to meats like chicken, tofu, or fish, marinate them in a mixture of ACV, olive oil, garlic, herbs, and spices.

Health-Conscious Recipes using ACV
Here are some health-conscious recipes that demonstrate the adaptability of ACV in salads and cooked dishes:

1. Kale salad with ACV dressing.

Ingredients:
- 1 bunch kale, stems removed, leaves finely sliced.
- 1/4 cup dried cranberries.
- 1/4 cup toasted almonds, chopped.

- 1/4 cup shredded Parmesan cheese (optional)
- ACV Dressing: 1/4 cup vinegar, 1/2 cup olive oil, 1 tablespoon honey, salt, and pepper.

Instructions:

- In a large bowl, massage kale leaves with olive oil until softened.
- Combine the dried cranberries, roasted almonds, and Parmesan cheese (if using).
- To prepare the dressing, combine the apple cider vinegar, olive oil, honey, salt, and pepper in a small bowl.
- Toss the salad with the dressing until it is evenly coated, then serve immediately.

2. ACV-Glazed Chicken

Ingredients:

- 4 boneless and skinless chicken breasts.
- 1/4 cup of raw, unfiltered ACV
- 2 tablespoons of honey.
- 1 tablespoon soy sauce (or tamari if gluten-free).
- 2 garlic cloves, minced
- Add salt and pepper to taste.

Instructions:

- In a mixing bowl, combine ACV, honey, soy sauce, minced garlic, salt, and pepper.
- Put the chicken breasts in a resealable plastic bag or shallow dish and pour the marinade over them.

- Seal or cover and chill for at least 30 minutes (up to 4 hours).
- Grill the chicken for 6-7 minutes per side, or until it is cooked through and the juices run clear, on a medium-high heat grill or grill pan.

Serve hot and garnish with fresh herbs if preferred

Integrating ACV into Various Culinary Preferences

Whether you adhere to a specific diet or have dietary preferences, ACV can be tailored to a variety of culinary styles:

Vegan and vegetarian diets: Use ACV in dressings, sauces, and marinades to add tangy flavor to plant-based foods while also potentially improving health.

Paleo & Keto Diets: ACV is naturally low in carbs and can be used sparingly to impart acidity to foods without drastically altering macronutrient ratios.

Gluten-Free and Dairy-Free Diets: Because ACV is naturally gluten-free and dairy-free, it is an adaptable component for individuals following dietary restrictions.

Tips for Choosing and Using ACV

To make the most of ACV in your culinary creations, consider the following tips:

Quality: Select high-quality, raw, unfiltered ACV with the mother for the most possible health benefits and flavor.

To keep ACV fresh and potent, store it in a cool, dark place or in the refrigerator after opening.

To balance the acidity and flavor of ACV, use it in moderation in salads, sauces, and marinades.

Safety considerations
While ACV is typically healthy for most people when used in culinary applications, moderation and consideration of individual health variables are required.

Dilution: To reduce throat or stomach irritation, dilute ACV with other ingredients such as oil, water, or citrus juice when using it in salads and sauces.

Allergic Reactions: Some people may be allergic to apples or develop allergic reactions to ACV; if you have any side effects, discontinue consumption and consult a doctor.

Incorporating ACV into salad dressings and sauces is not only a delicious way to enhance flavors, but also a practical approach to potentially supporting overall health and well-being. Whether you're looking to boost digestion, regulate blood sugar levels, or simply enjoy vibrant and nutritious meals, ACV has versatility and health benefits that can elevate your culinary experiences.

By experimenting with different recipes, using seasonal ingredients, and incorporating ACV into your daily cooking routine, you can discover a world of flavors and health-conscious choices. Embrace the tangy goodness of apple cider vinegar and enjoy the transformative power it brings to your salads, sauces, and more.

Chapter 5

Enhancing Meat and Vegetarian Options with Apple Cider Vinegar

Apple cider vinegar (ACV) is a versatile ingredient that can improve the flavor and nutritional profile of main dishes, whether you're preparing meat-based recipes or exploring vegetarian and vegan options. ACV's tangy acidity and potential health benefits make it a valuable addition to a wide range of culinary creations, from hearty stews and marinades to vibrant vegetable dishes and sauces. In this comprehensive guide, we'll explore

- Understanding ACV's Role in Main Dishes

ACV is made from fermented apple cider and has a sharp, tangy flavor due to its acetic acid content. When used in main dishes, ACV not only adds a distinctive taste but also contributes to tenderizing meats, balancing flavors, and potentially offering health benefits. Here's how ACV plays a role in both meat and vegetarian main dishes.

- Mechanism and Health Benefits

Flavor Enhancement: ACV's acidity brightens and balances flavors in marinades and sauces, improving the overall taste of foods without overpowering other components.

Tenderizing Agent: ACV's acidic nature can tenderize meat by breaking down muscle fibers, resulting in more tender and tasty cuts when used in marinades or braising liquids.

Potential Digestive Support: According to some research, ACV may improve digestion by increasing the synthesis of digestive enzymes and supporting a healthy gut environment, which can be beneficial independent of dietary preferences.

Health Advantages of Using ACV in Main Dishes
Incorporating ACV into main courses has various possible health benefits:

Digestive improve: ACV's acidity may improve digestion by increasing stomach acid production, thereby improving nutrient absorption and relieving digestive discomfort.

Blood Sugar Regulation: According to preliminary studies, ACV may help enhance insulin sensitivity and lower blood sugar levels after high-carbohydrate meals, making it a useful supplement for people who need to manage their blood sugar levels.

ACV contains antioxidants such as polyphenols, which can help counteract oxidative stress and free radical damage, promoting overall cellular health and potentially lowering the risk of chronic disease.

- Practical Tips for Cooking with ACV

Whether you're making meat-based dishes or looking into vegetarian options, here are some practical ideas for adding ACV into your cooking:

1. Marinades for meat and tofu
ACV-based marinades can improve the flavor and tenderness of meats and tofu.

Basic marinade recipe:

- Ingredients: 1/4 cup ACV, 1/4 cup olive oil, 2 cloves minced garlic, 1 tablespoon honey or maple syrup, salt, and pepper.
- Marinate meat or tofu in a mixture of apple cider vinegar, olive oil, garlic, honey or maple syrup, salt, and pepper for at least 30 minutes (or up to overnight) before cooking.

2. Sauces and glazes.
ACV can be used to make excellent sauces and glazes for meats, veggies, and grains.

BBQ Sauce: Mix ACV with tomato paste, honey, Worcestershire sauce, and spices to make a tangy BBQ sauce that goes well with grilled chicken, ribs, or tofu.

Pan Sauce: After cooking meat or veggies in a skillet, deglaze with ACV and broth, then reduce to make a tasty pan sauce. Season with herbs and spices as desired.

3. Salad dressings.

ACV-based salad dressings are a versatile topping for both meat and vegetarian main entrees.

Balsamic Vinaigrette: Combine ACV, balsamic vinegar, olive oil, Dijon mustard, and honey to make a classic dressing that goes well with grilled meats, roasted vegetables, and salads.

Citrus Dressing: Make a vibrant and tangy dressing with ACV, freshly squeezed citrus juice (such as lemon or lime), olive oil, garlic, and herbs. Serve over seafood or mixed greens.

- Recipes with ACV in main dishes

Discover these tasty and healthful recipes that highlight ACV's adaptability in both meat-based and vegetarian main courses.

1. ACV-Braised Pork Shoulder

Ingredients:

- 3-4 pounds of pork shoulder, bone-in
- 1/2 cup of raw, unfiltered ACV
- 1/4 cup low-sodium soy sauce (tamari for gluten-free)
- 2 tablespoons of honey.
- 4 garlic cloves, minced
- One onion, sliced
- 2 cups of chicken or vegetarian broth.
- Add salt and pepper to taste.

Instructions:

- Preheat the oven to 325° F (165° C).

- Season the pork shoulder with salt and pepper.
- In a Dutch oven or large oven-safe pot, heat olive oil over medium-high heat and sear the pork shoulder on all sides until browned, about 6-8 minutes total.
- Remove the pork from the saucepan and set it aside. Sauté the onions and garlic in the pot until they're tender and aromatic.
- Deglaze the pot with ACV and soy sauce, scraping out any browned bits on the bottom.
- Return the pork shoulder to the pot, along with the honey and broth; bring to a simmer.
- Cover and bake for 2.5 to 3 hours, or until the pork is soft and readily separated with a fork.
- Serve hot and garnish with fresh herbs if preferred.

2. ACV Roasted Brussels sprouts
Ingredients:

- 1 pound of Brussels sprouts, cut and halved
- 2 tablespoons of olive oil.
- 2 teaspoons of raw, unfiltered ACV
- 1 tablespoon honey.
- Add salt and pepper to taste.

Instructions:

- Preheat the oven to 400° F (200° C).
- Toss Brussels sprouts in a large bowl with olive oil, apple cider vinegar, honey, salt, and pepper until equally covered.

- Spread the Brussels sprouts in a single layer on a baking sheet.
- Roast for 20-25 minutes, tossing halfway, or until the Brussels sprouts are soft and caramelized.
- Serve hot as a side dish, or mix into grain bowls or salads.

Integrating ACV into Various Culinary Preferences

ACV can be tailored to suit a variety of dietary choices and culinary styles.

Vegan and vegetarian diets: Add ACV to marinades, sauces, and dressings for tofu, tempeh, and vegetable dishes to improve flavor and texture.

Paleo & Keto Diets: ACV is naturally low in carbs and can be used sparingly to impart acidity to foods without drastically altering macronutrient ratios.

Gluten-Free and Dairy-Free Diets: Because ACV is naturally gluten-free and dairy-free, it is an adaptable component for individuals following dietary restrictions.

Tips for Selecting and Using ACV in Main Dishes

To make the most of ACV in your main dish dishes, consider the following suggestions:

Choose high-quality, raw, unfiltered ACV with the mother for the best flavor and potential health benefits.

Balance: Use ACV sparingly to balance its acidity and ensure that it complements other elements in your recipes.

Experimentation: Don't be hesitant to try different types and amounts of ACV to find the flavor profile that works best for your palate and dish.

Safety considerations
While ACV is typically healthy for most people when used in culinary applications, moderation and consideration of individual health variables are required.

Dilution: When using ACV in marinades, sauces, or dressings, always dilute it with oil, broth, or citrus juice to avoid throat and stomach irritation.

Allergic Reactions: Some people may be allergic to apples or develop allergic reactions to ACV; if you have any side effects, discontinue consumption and consult a doctor.

Incorporating ACV into main dishes offers a flavorful and potentially health-promoting addition to your culinary repertoire, whether you're preparing meat-based recipes or exploring vegetarian and vegan options. The versatility of ACV makes it a valuable ingredient in a variety of dishes, from tenderizing meats and enhancing flavors to supporting digestion and possibly regulating blood sugar levels.

By experimenting with different recipes, embracing seasonal ingredients, and incorporating ACV into your daily cooking routine, you can elevate your meals with tangy goodness and health-conscious choices. Accept the versatility of apple cider vinegar and enjoy the transformative power it brings to your main dishes, enhancing both taste and potential health benefits for you and your loved ones.

Chapter 6

ACV in Baking and Desserts: Adding Flavor, Texture, and Possible Health Benefits

Apple cider vinegar (ACV) is a versatile ingredient that can enhance the flavor, texture, and even the nutritional profile of baked goods and desserts. With its tangy acidity and potential health benefits, ACV adds a unique twist to everything from cakes and cookies to bread and sauces. In this comprehensive guide, we'll explore how ACV can be used effectively in baking and desserts, discuss its role in enhancing

Understanding the role of ACV in baking and desserts
ACV is derived from fermented apple cider and includes acetic acid, which gives it its characteristic tangy flavor and potential health-promoting effects. In baking and sweets, ACV performs a variety of functions, including

Leavening Agent: When coupled with baking soda, ACV causes a chemical reaction that produces carbon dioxide gas, allowing baked goods to rise and become lighter and fluffy.
Flavor Enhancer: ACV provides a delicate sour flavor that compliments sweet ingredients and balances the overall taste of desserts.

Tenderizer: ACV's acidic nature can help tenderize gluten in baked foods, resulting in softer textures.

Health Advantages of Using ACV in Baking and Desserts

Incorporating ACV into baking and pastries may provide possible health benefits:

Digestive Aid: The acidity of ACV may increase the production of stomach acid, improving digestion and maybe reducing bloating or discomfort after meals.

Blood Sugar Regulation: According to some research, ACV can help enhance insulin sensitivity and lower blood sugar levels, making it useful for people who need to manage their blood glucose levels.

Antioxidant Properties: ACV contains antioxidants like polyphenols, which can help neutralize free radicals and minimize oxidative stress in the body, potentially improving general health.

Practical Tips for Baking with ACV

Baking with ACV is simple and may be included into a number of recipes. Here are some useful things to consider:

1. Leavening with ACV and baking soda

Here's how to use ACV as a leavening agent:

Ingredients:

- 1 teaspoon of baking soda.
- 1 tablespoon of raw, unfiltered ACV
- Instructions:
- In a small bowl or measuring cup, combine baking soda and apple cider vinegar.
- Gently stir until the mixture starts to froth and bubble.

- Incorporate immediately into your batter or dough, mixing thoroughly to ensure that the leavening activity is uniformly distributed.

2. ACV substitutes for other acids

In many recipes, ACV can be replaced for other acids such as lemon juice or buttermilk.

- To make a buttermilk substitute, mix 1 cup of milk with 1 tablespoon of apple cider vinegar or lemon juice and let it sit for a few minutes until it curdles before using.

3. Enhanced Flavor Profiles

Experiment with various types of ACV to improve the flavor profiles in your baked goods:

Raw vs. Filtered ACV: Raw, unfiltered ACV with the mother intact has a stronger flavor and potential health advantages than filtered ACV.

Infused ACV: To add subtle fragrant notes to your baking, soak herbs or spices in ACV for several days before use.

Recipes with ACV in Baking and Desserts

Discover these delectable recipes that demonstrate ACV's adaptability and potential in baking and sweets.

1. Classic ACV Chocolate Cake.
Ingredients:

- 1 3/4 cups all-purpose flour.
- 1 cup granulated sugar.
- 1/2 cup cocoa powder.
- 1 teaspoon of baking powder.
- 1 teaspoon of baking soda.
- 1/2 teaspoon of salt.
- 1 cup water.
- 1/2 cup vegetable oil.
- 1 tablespoon of raw, unfiltered ACV
- 1 teaspoon of vanilla extract.

Instructions:

- Preheat the oven to 350°F (175°C). Grease and flour a 9x9-inch baking pan.
- In a large bowl, combine the flour, sugar, cocoa powder, baking powder, baking soda, and salt.
- In a separate bowl, combine the water, vegetable oil, ACV, and vanilla essence.
- Pour the wet ingredients into the dry ingredients and mix just until mixed.
- Pour the batter into the prepared pan, smoothing the top.
- Bake for 25–30 minutes, or until a toothpick inserted in the center comes out clean.
- Let cool completely on a wire rack before icing or serving.

2. ACV Apple Cinnamon Muffins.
Ingredients:

- 2 cups of all-purpose flour.

- 1/2 cup granulated sugar.
- 2 tablespoons baking powder.
- 1/2 teaspoon of baking soda.
- 1/2 teaspoon of salt.
- 1 teaspoon ground cinnamon.
- 1/4 cup melted butter or vegetable oil.
- 1/2 cup applesauce.
- 1/2 cup milk (or non-dairy milk).
- 2 teaspoons of raw, unfiltered ACV
- 1 teaspoon of vanilla extract.
- 1 cup diced apples.

Instructions:

- Preheat the oven to 375°F (190°C). Line a muffin tray with paper liners or oil thoroughly.
- In a large basin, combine the flour, sugar, baking powder, baking soda, salt, and cinnamon.
- In a separate bowl, add the melted butter or oil, applesauce, milk, ACV, and vanilla extract.
- Pour wet ingredients into dry ingredients and whisk until just incorporated, then fold in diced apples.
- Spoon batter into prepared muffin cups, filling them approximately 3/4 full.
- Bake for 18 to 20 minutes, or until a toothpick inserted in the center comes out clean.
- Cool in the pan for 5 minutes before transferring to a wire rack to cool fully.

Integrating ACV into Various Dietary Preferences

ACV can be tailored to meet a variety of dietary choices and constraints.

Vegan and vegetarian diets: ACV can be used as a leavening agent, flavor enhancer, or substitution for dairy-based products in vegan baking recipes.

Gluten-Free Diets: ACV is naturally gluten-free and can be used in gluten-free baking recipes to improve texture and flavor.

Paleo and Keto Diets: Use ACV sparingly in paleo and keto baking recipes, and adjust other ingredients to maintain macronutrient ratios.

Tips for Selecting and Using ACV in Baking and Desserts
To optimize the advantages of ACV in your baking and pastries, consider the following:

Choose high-quality, raw, unfiltered ACV with the mother for the best flavor and potential health benefits.

Measurement: When using ACV as a leavening agent, follow the recipe exactly to ensure the right component balance and the desired texture.

Experimentation: Don't be afraid to try different types and quantities of ACV to find the flavor profile that works best for your baking creations.

Safety considerations

While ACV is typically healthy for most people when used in culinary applications, moderation and consideration of individual health variables are required.

Dilution: To avoid throat or stomach irritation, always dilute ACV with water, milk, or oil while baking.

Allergic Reactions: Some people may be allergic to apples or develop allergic reactions to ACV; if you have any side effects, discontinue consumption and consult a doctor.

Incorporating ACV into baking and desserts provides a delectable and potentially health-enhancing addition to your culinary repertoire. Whether you're making cakes, muffins, bread, or experimenting with sauces and glazes, ACV can provide a unique twist with its sour flavor and potential health benefits.

By experimenting with different recipes, adapting to dietary preferences, and using apple cider vinegar mindfully in your baking endeavors, you can create delicious treats that not only satisfy your taste buds but also contribute to your overall well-being. Accept the versatility of apple cider vinegar and enjoy the transformative impact it brings to your favorite baked goods and desserts, making every bite a delightful and nutritious experience.

Chapter 7

Beauty and Skincare Recipes with Apple Cider Vinegar (ACV): Using Natural Benefits for Radiant Skin and Hair

Apple cider vinegar (ACV) has gained popularity not only in the realm of culinary use but also in the realm of beauty and skincare due to its potential natural benefits. Known for its acidic nature and nutrient content, ACV is celebrated for its ability to balance pH levels, exfoliate, tone, and clarify skin and hair. In this comprehensive guide, we will explore the science behind ACV's skin care benefits, delve into various beauty recipes, and discuss its application for different skin types.

Understanding the benefits of ACV for the skin and hair

Apple cider vinegar (ACV) is a strong elixir that contains acetic acid, vitamins (such as vitamin C and B), minerals, and enzymes, all of which contribute to ACV's potential beauty and skincare advantages.

- Mechanism and Properties

ACV is mildly acidic, similar to the skin's natural pH, which aids in the restoration and maintenance of the skin's acid mantle. This balance is essential for good skin function and protection against environmental stresses.

Exfoliation: ACV's natural acids, including acetic acid, gently exfoliate the skin, eliminating dead skin cells and boosting cell turnover, resulting in smoother, brighter skin.

Antibacterial and antifungal properties: ACV includes antimicrobial components that can help treat bacteria and fungi on the skin, potentially lowering the risk of acne and other skin problems.

Toning and Clarifying: ACV is a natural astringent that tightens pores and refines skin texture. It can also clear the complexion by removing excess oil and pollutants.

Health Advantages of Using ACV in Beauty and Skincare
Adding ACV to your cosmetic routine can provide various potential health benefits for your skin and hair:

Acne Control: ACV's antibacterial characteristics may aid in the reduction of acne-causing germs and the regulation of oil production, potentially reducing outbreaks.

Skin Brightening: Regular application of ACV can help exfoliate dull skin, revealing a more radiant complexion over time.

Scalp Health: ACV can balance scalp pH, relieve itching, and reduce dandruff by restoring natural oils and maintaining a healthy microbial balance.

- Practical Advice for Using ACV in Beauty and Skincare

When using ACV in beauty and skincare routines, consider the following suggestions for safe and effective use:

1. Dilution and Application.
ACV is highly acidic, thus it should always be diluted with water or other components before applying to the skin or hair.

To make a facial toner, combine one part apple cider vinegar and three parts water, then apply to cleansed skin with a cotton pad or spritz. Follow with moisturizer.

Hair Rinse: After shampooing, dilute ACV with water in a 1:1 ratio and apply to your hair and scalp. Massage gently and completely rinse with water.

2. Patch Testing.
Before using ACV-based treatments on wider regions of skin or hair, perform a patch test to check for any adverse reactions.

Apply a little amount of diluted ACV to a discrete region of skin (such as the inner forearm) and wait 24 hours. If there is no irritation, the product is safe to use.

3. Frequency
Begin by using ACV treatments once or twice a week to see how your skin and hair react; then, adjust the frequency based on your skin's tolerance and desired outcomes.

- Beauty and Skincare Recipes using ACV

Explore these powerful and simple beauty recipes that use apple cider vinegar to achieve beautiful skin and healthy hair.

1. ACV Clarifying Facial Toner.
Ingredients:

- 1/4 cup of raw, unfiltered ACV
- 3/4 cup purified water.
- 5-10 drops of essential oil (optional: lavender or tea tree)

Instructions:

- In a small bowl or container, combine ACV and water.
- If desired, add essential oil to enhance the benefits and scent.
- Shake thoroughly before each usage.
- Apply to cleansed skin with a cotton pad as a toner, avoiding the eye area.
- Apply moisturizer daily or as needed.

2. ACV Hair Rinse Promotes Scalp Health
Ingredients:

- 1/2 cup of raw, unfiltered ACV
- 1/2 cup water.

Instructions:

- In a bowl, combine the ACV and water.

- After shampooing, apply the mixture to damp hair and scalp.
- Massage lightly into your scalp for a few minutes.
- Rinse well with water.
- Use once each week to keep your scalp healthy and reduce dandruff.

Integrating ACV into Various Skincare Needs

ACV can be used to treat a variety of skincare issues and conditions.

Acne-Prone Skin: Apply ACV as a spot treatment for acne or as a toner to balance oil production and prevent outbreaks.

For sensitive skin, dilute ACV further and use it less frequently to decrease irritation. You may also combine it with calming substances like aloe vera or chamomile.

Dry or mature skin: Add ACV to moisturizing masks or moisturizers to gently exfoliate and enhance skin texture without overdrying.

Tips for Selecting ACV for Beauty and Skincare

To get the most out of ACV in your beauty routine, consider the following guidelines while selecting and utilizing it:

Choose raw, unfiltered ACV with the "mother" for optimum potency and potential benefits.

To keep ACV effective over time, store it in a cool, dark spot away from direct sunlight.

Organic Options: When feasible, use organic ACV to reduce your exposure to pesticides and other toxins.

Safety considerations

While ACV is typically safe for topical usage, it's important to be cautious and monitor your skin's reaction.

Avoid Undiluted Use: Never apply undiluted ACV to your skin or scalp because it might irritate or burn.

Consultation: If you have sensitive skin or underlying skin concerns, talk to a specialist before introducing ACV into your skincare program.

Incorporating ACV into your beauty and skincare regimen offers a natural and effective way to enhance skin and hair health. Whether you're looking to clarify your complexion, balance oily skin, or improve scalp conditions, ACV provides a versatile solution due to its acidic properties and nutrient-rich composition.

By experimenting with DIY recipes, adjusting formulations to suit your skin type, and incorporating ACV into your regular skincare routine, you can harness its potential benefits for radiant, healthy skin and hair. Embrace the power of apple cider vinegar and discover the transformative effects it can bring to your beauty regimen, making each application a step toward natural beauty and wellness.

Chapter 8

ACV for Digestive Health: Using Nature's Remedy for Gut Wellness and More

Apple cider vinegar (ACV) has long been hailed for its potential to improve digestive health. ACV is well-known for its inherent acidity and nutritional profile, which aids digestion and nutrient absorption while also promoting gut flora balance. In this comprehensive guide, we will look at the science behind ACV's digestive advantages, its possible applications, its function in gut health, practical recommendations for incorporating ACV into your diet, and a number of recipes and cures to support digestive wellness.

Understanding the Benefits of ACV for Digestive Health

ACV is made by fermenting apple cider, which produces a strong elixir high in acetic acid, enzymes, probiotics, and prebiotics. These components contribute to ACV's possible digestive health advantages.

- Mechanism and Properties

Aiding Digestion: ACV's acidity may encourage the generation of stomach acid (hydrochloric acid), which is necessary for food breakdown and nutrient absorption.

Supporting Gut Microbiota: ACV's probiotics and prebiotics may help maintain a healthy balance of gut flora, boosting overall digestive wellness.

Alleviating Digestive Discomfort: The enzymes and nutrients in ACV can help with digestion and relieve symptoms such as bloating, gas, and indigestion.

- Health Advantages of Using ACV for Digestive Health:

Adding ACV to your diet may provide numerous potential health benefits for digestive wellness:

Improved Digestion: The acidity in ACV can help with digestion, potentially reducing bloating and discomfort after meals.

Contrary to popular opinion, ACV may help regulate stomach acid levels, hence assisting people with low stomach acid (hypochlorhydria).

Gut Microbiota Support: Probiotics in ACV may help to maintain a healthy gut environment, which is essential for immune function, nutrition absorption, and overall well-being.

- Practical Guidelines for Using ACV for Digestive Health

When introducing ACV into your diet for digestive health, consider these useful guidelines for safe and efficient use:

1. Dilution and Consumption

ACV is highly acidic, thus it should be diluted with water or other liquids before intake.

ACV Tonic: Combine 1-2 tablespoons of ACV and 8-10 ounces of water. If desired, flavor with honey or lemon juice.

Salad Dressing: Use ACV as a base for homemade salad dressings to reap its digestive benefits while also adding flavor to your food.

2. Timing and frequency
Begin with tiny doses of ACV and progressively increase according to your tolerance and digestive response.

Morning Routine: Add ACV to your morning routine by drinking a diluted tonic on an empty stomach to stimulate digestion.

Before Meals: Drink a little amount of diluted ACV to aid digestion and improve nutrient absorption.

- Recipes with ACV for Digestive Health

Discover these nutritious and delicious dishes that use ACV to promote digestive health:

1. ACV Ginger Digestive Tonic.
Ingredients:

- 1 tablespoon of raw, unfiltered ACV
- 1 teaspoon of freshly grated ginger.
- One tablespoon honey (optional)
- 8-10 ounces of warm water.

Instructions:

- In a mug, mix the ACV, grated ginger, and honey (if using).
- Pour warm water over the mixture and whisk thoroughly.
- Drink carefully before or between meals to help digestion and soothe the stomach.

2. ACV and Honey Dressing

Ingredients:

- 1/4 cup of raw, unfiltered ACV
- 1/4 cup extra virgin olive oil.
- 1 tablespoon honey.
- 1 teaspoon Dijon mustard.
- Add salt and pepper to taste.

Instructions:

- In a small mixing bowl, add ACV, olive oil, honey, Dijon mustard, salt, and pepper until well blended.
- Drizzle over salads or marinate meats to add taste and aid digestion.

Integrating ACV into Various Dietary Preferences
ACV can be tailored to meet a variety of dietary tastes and demands.

Vegan and vegetarian diets: Use ACV in dressings, marinades, and tonics to add flavor and digestive assistance without using animal products.

Paleo & Keto Diets: ACV is naturally low in carbs and can be used sparingly to impart acidity to meals without changing macronutrient ratios.

Gluten-Free and Dairy-Free Diets: ACV is naturally gluten-free and dairy-free, making it acceptable for people who have dietary limitations.

Tips for Selecting ACV for Digestive Health
To maximize the benefits of ACV for digestive health, consider the following tips:

Choose raw, unfiltered ACV with the "mother" for optimum potency and potential health benefits.

Organic Options: Choose organic ACV wherever possible to reduce your exposure to pesticides and other toxins.

To maintain ACV's quality and effectiveness, store it in a cool, dark place away from direct sunlight.

- Safety considerations

While ACV is generally safe for most individuals when consumed in moderation, it is critical to exercise caution and monitor your body's response.

To avoid irritating the throat or stomach lining, always dilute ACV with water or other drinks.

Sensitive Stomachs: If you have a history of gastrointestinal troubles or sensitivities, begin with tiny doses of ACV and monitor your body's reaction.

Incorporating ACV into your diet for digestive health is a natural and efficient way to promote overall well-being. Whether you use it as a morning tonic, in salad dressings, or as a meat marinade, ACV offers a varied solution due to its acidic qualities and potential digestive advantages.

Experiment with different recipes, alter formulations to your taste preferences, and incorporate ACV into your normal diet to reap its potential advantages for digestive health and overall well-being. Accept the power of apple cider vinegar and learn how it can benefit your digestive system, making each drink and bite a step toward a healthier, happier you.

Chapter 9

ACV for Weight Management: Investigating Its Role in Promoting Healthy Weight Loss and Maintenance

Apple cider vinegar (ACV) has grown in favor as a natural weight-loss solution due to its possible effects on metabolism, hunger regulation, and blood sugar levels. ACV, which is made from fermented apple cider, is high in acetic acid and nutrients and may provide a variety of benefits to people seeking to achieve and maintain a healthy weight. In this comprehensive guide, we will look at the science behind ACV's potential for weight management, investigate its mechanisms of action, discuss practical ways to incorporate ACV into your diet, and provide evidence-based insights and tips to help you use ACV effectively in your weight loss journey.

- Understanding the Potential of ACV for Weight Management.

ACV is thought to affect weight management by a variety of ways, including:

1. Regulation of Blood Sugar Levels

ACV may help to maintain blood sugar levels by increasing insulin sensitivity and lowering blood sugar increases after meals. This could potentially reduce insulin levels, which are linked to fat accumulation and weight growth.

2. Appetite Suppression

The acetic acid in ACV has been demonstrated to promote sensations of fullness and satiety, resulting in decreased calorie intake throughout the day. This can help you avoid overeating and support your weight loss goals.

3. Metabolism Boost

Some research indicates that ACV may improve metabolism, perhaps improving the pace at which the body burns calories and fat. When combined with a balanced diet and lifestyle, this impact may contribute to long-term weight loss.

- Health Advantages of Using ACV for Weight Management

Adding ACV to your diet may provide various potential health benefits connected to weight management:

Supports Healthy Metabolism: ACV's effect on metabolism may aid in weight loss by increasing calorie expenditure.

Increases Satiety: Because ACV increases sensations of fullness, it can help you eat less and control your appetite.

ACV can help control blood sugar levels by boosting insulin sensitivity, which may reduce cravings and promote fat burning.

- Practical Guidelines for Using ACV for Weight Management

When utilizing ACV for weight management, consider these practical steps to maximize its advantages.

1. Dilution and Consumption
ACV is highly acidic, thus it should be diluted with water or other liquids before intake.

ACV Tonic: Combine 1-2 tablespoons of ACV and 8-10 ounces of water. If desired, flavor with honey or lemon juice. Drink this tonic before meals to improve digestion and hunger management.

Salad Dressing: Use ACV as a foundation for homemade salad dressings to boost flavor and satiety during meals.

2. Timing and frequency
Incorporate ACV into your regular routine to help weight management goals.

Morning Routine: Begin the day with an ACV tonic to boost metabolism and induce satiety throughout the morning.

Before Meals: Take a tiny amount of diluted ACV before meals to help reduce hunger and blood sugar levels.

- Evidence-Based Insights on ACV for Weight Management
While ACV has promise for weight management, it is important to understand its limitations and implications.

Limited Research: The majority of studies on ACV's benefits on weight management are tiny and short-term. More study is needed to determine the long-term benefits and ideal dosages.

Individual Variability: The effects of ACV can differ between individuals depending on factors like as diet, genetics, and overall health.

For best weight control benefits, ACV should be used in conjunction with a well-balanced diet and a healthy lifestyle that includes frequent exercise and proper sleep.

- Recipes using ACV for Weight Management

Explore these nutritious and enjoyable dishes with ACV to support your weight loss goals:

1. ACV detox drink

Ingredients:

- 1 tablespoon of raw, unfiltered ACV
- Juice from 1/2 lemon
- 1 teaspoon of grated ginger.
- One tablespoon honey (optional)
- 8-10 ounces of warm water.

Instructions:

- In a mug, mix the ACV, lemon juice, grated ginger, and honey (if using).
- Pour warm water over the mixture and whisk thoroughly.
- This detox tonic should be taken on an empty stomach in the morning to enhance cleansing and metabolism.

2. ACV-Grilled Chicken Salad

Ingredients:

- 2 boneless and skinless chicken breasts.
- Add salt and pepper to taste.
- 2 teaspoons of raw, unfiltered ACV
- 1 tablespoon of olive oil.
- Mixed salad greens.
- Cherry tomatoes, sliced cucumber, and other salad vegetables of your choice

Instructions:

- Season the chicken breasts with salt and pepper.
- In a small bowl, combine ACV and olive oil to make a marinade.
- Marinate chicken breasts in this mixture for at least 30 minutes.
- Grill or grill chicken breasts until well done and the juices flow clear.
- Slice the chicken and serve over mixed salad greens with cherry tomatoes, cucumber, and other vegetables. Drizzle with more ACV dressing if desired.

Integrating ACV into Various Dietary Preferences

ACV can be tailored to meet a variety of dietary tastes and demands.

Vegan and vegetarian diets: Use ACV in dressings, marinades, and tonics to provide taste and fullness without using animal products.

Paleo & Keto Diets: ACV is naturally low in carbs and can be used sparingly to impart acidity to meals without changing macronutrient ratios.

Gluten-Free and Dairy-Free Diets: ACV is naturally gluten-free and dairy-free, making it acceptable for people who have dietary limitations.

Tips for Selecting ACV for Weight Management
To get the most out of ACV for weight management, consider these suggestions while choosing and utilizing it:

Choose raw, unfiltered ACV with the "mother" for optimum potency and potential health benefits.

Organic Options: Choose organic ACV wherever possible to reduce your exposure to pesticides and other toxins.

To maintain ACV's quality and effectiveness, store it in a cool, dark place away from direct sunlight.

Safety considerations
While ACV is generally safe for most individuals when consumed in moderation, it is critical to exercise caution and monitor your body's response.

To avoid irritating the throat or stomach lining, always dilute ACV with water or other drinks.

Sensitive Stomachs: If you have a history of gastrointestinal troubles or sensitivities, begin with tiny doses of ACV and monitor your body's reaction.

Incorporating ACV into your diet for weight control is a natural and potentially beneficial way to assist healthy weight loss and maintenance. Whether you drink it as a morning tonic, use it as a salad dressing base, or include it into savory foods, ACV offers a diverse option due to its acidic qualities and potential metabolic benefits.

By including ACV into your daily routine and supplementing it with a healthy diet and frequent physical activity, you can reap its potential advantages for weight control and overall well-being. Accept the power of apple cider vinegar and learn how it can help you achieve a better weight, making each meal and sip a step toward a more energetic and balanced living.

Chapter 10

Exploring the Potential Benefits of ACV for Energy and Immunity

Apple cider vinegar (ACV) has been identified not just for its culinary applications, but also for its potential health advantages, such as increasing energy and immunological function. ACV, made from fermented apple cider, has a number of minerals and bioactive components that contribute to its claimed effects on energy metabolism and immunological response. In this comprehensive guide, we will look at the science behind ACV's potential energy and immunity benefits, as well as its mechanisms of action. We will also discuss practical ways to incorporate ACV into your daily routine and provide evidence-based insights and tips to help you maximize its effects on vitality.

- Understanding ACV's Potential for Energy and Immunity

ACV is thought to affect energy levels and immunological function via numerous pathways, including:

1. Nutrient Content
ACV is high in vitamins (particularly vitamin C and B vitamins), minerals (such as potassium), enzymes, and antioxidants, all of which are necessary for energy production and immune support.

2. Metabolism Boost

Acetic acid in ACV may help with metabolism by boosting fat breakdown and enhancing insulin sensitivity, which can contribute to long-term energy levels.

3. Immune Modulation
ACV's antibacterial qualities and potential prebiotic benefits may aid in the maintenance of a healthy gut flora, which is critical for immune function and overall wellness.

- Health Advantages of Using ACV for Energy and Immunity

Incorporating ACV into your daily routine may provide various possible health benefits, including increased energy and immune support.

Increased Vitality: Because ACV improves metabolism and food absorption, it may help you feel more energized and vibrant.

Enhanced immunological Response: ACV's nutrients and bioactive components may help enhance immunological defenses and improve the body's ability to fight infections.

- Practical Guidelines for Using ACV for Energy and Immunity

When taking ACV to boost energy and promote immunological health, follow these practical tips to maximize its benefits:

1. Dilution and Consumption
ACV is highly acidic, thus it should be diluted with water or other liquids before intake.

ACV Tonic: Combine 1-2 tablespoons of ACV and 8-10 ounces of water. If desired, flavor with honey or lemon juice. Drink this tonic every day or as needed to boost energy and immunity.

Smoothies: Mix a dash of ACV into your favorite smoothie recipes to make a healthful and delicious drink.

2. Timing and frequency
Add ACV to your daily routine to maintain stable energy levels and improve immunological function.

Morning Routine: Begin the day with an ACV tonic to boost metabolism and general energy.

Throughout the Day: Drink diluted ACV water or mix it with meals and snacks to stay hydrated and improve digestive health.

- Evidence-Based Perspectives on ACV for Energy and Immunity.

While ACV shows potential for boosting energy and immunity, it's important to note the following evidence-based insights:

Metabolic Effects: Research suggests that ACV may enhance insulin sensitivity and lower blood sugar levels after meals, allowing for more sustained energy levels.

Antimicrobial Properties: ACV's antimicrobial activities may assist to restrict the growth of dangerous bacteria and promote a healthy gut microbiota, which is necessary for immunological function.

Nutrient Absorption: The enzymes and acids in ACV may help with nutrient absorption, ensuring that critical vitamins and minerals are used to produce energy and maintain immunological health.

- Recipes using ACV for Energy and Immunity.

Explore these healthful and delicious dishes that include ACV to increase energy and immune function:

1. ACV Citrus Energy Drink.
Ingredients:

- 1 tablespoon of raw, unfiltered ACV
- Juice from 1/2 lemon
- Juice from 1/2 orange
- One teaspoon honey (optional)
- 8-10 ounces of cold water.

Instructions:

- In a glass, combine the ACV, lemon juice, orange juice, and honey (if desired).
- Stir thoroughly until the honey has dissolved.
- Add cold water and stir completely.
- This delightful citrus energy drink is ideal for a midday pick-me-up.

2. ACV Immune-Boosting Salad Dressing
Ingredients:

- 1/4 cup of raw, unfiltered ACV

- 1/4 cup extra virgin olive oil.
- 1 tablespoon Dijon mustard.
- 1 teaspoon honey.
- 1 clove garlic, minced
- Add salt and pepper to taste.

Instructions:

- In a small mixing bowl, blend ACV, olive oil, Dijon mustard, honey, minced garlic, salt, and pepper until well incorporated.
- Drizzle over mixed greens and vegetables, or marinate grilled chicken or tofu.
- Enjoy this immune-boosting salad dressing to improve overall health and wellness.

Integrating ACV into Various Dietary Preferences

ACV can be tailored to meet a variety of dietary tastes and demands.

Vegan and vegetarian diets: Use ACV in dressings, marinades, and tonics to improve flavor and nutritional absorption without using animal products.

Paleo & Keto Diets: ACV is naturally low in carbs and can be used sparingly to impart acidity to meals without changing macronutrient ratios.

Gluten-Free and Dairy-Free Diets: ACV is naturally gluten-free and dairy-free, making it acceptable for people who have dietary limitations.

Tips for Selecting ACV for Energy and Immunity
To get the most out of ACV for energy and immunological support, consider the following guidelines while selecting and using it:

Choose raw, unfiltered ACV with the "mother" for optimum potency and potential health benefits.

Organic Options: Choose organic ACV wherever possible to reduce your exposure to pesticides and other toxins.

To maintain ACV's quality and effectiveness, store it in a cool, dark place away from direct sunlight.

Safety considerations
While ACV is generally safe for most individuals when consumed in moderation, it is critical to exercise caution and monitor your body's response.

To avoid irritating the throat or stomach lining, always dilute ACV with water or other drinks.

Individuals with a history of gastrointestinal difficulties or sensitivities should start with minimal doses of ACV and observe how their bodies react.

Incorporating ACV into your daily routine to boost energy and immunity is a natural and potentially effective strategy to promote overall vitality and wellness. Whether you drink it as a refreshing tonic, add it into your favorite dishes, or use it as a salad dressing base, ACV offers a diverse option due to its acidic qualities and potential health advantages.

You may get the benefits of ACV for energy and immune support by incorporating it into your diet and lifestyle, in addition to a balanced diet, frequent exercise, and adequate rest. Accept the power of apple cider vinegar and learn how it can help you achieve optimal vitality and wellness, with each drink and bite bringing you closer to a healthier and more vibrant you.

Chapter 11

Safety Tips and Precautions for Using Apple Cider Vinegar (ACV): Ensure Safe and Effective Use

Apple cider vinegar (ACV) has grown in popularity due to its possible health benefits, which include digestive support and weight management. However, like any natural medicine, ACV should be used with caution to avoid any side effects. In this comprehensive guide, we will look at the safety concerns surrounding ACV, examine potential risks and precautions, provide practical suggestions for safe use, and present evidence-based insights to help you integrate ACV into your lifestyle responsibly.

- Understanding the composition and applications of ACV
ACV is manufactured by fermenting apple cider, which produces vinegar that maintains many of the beneficial elements contained in apples. Acetic acid, vitamins (including vitamin C and B), minerals (such as potassium), enzymes, and polyphenols are all important components of ACV. These components contribute to its potential health advantages, but they also require cautious caution when using ACV.

- Potential risks and considerations.

While ACV is typically safe for most individuals when used correctly, there are a few potential hazards and precautions to be aware of:

1. Acetic Acid Content

ACV is extremely acidic due to its acetic acid concentration, which can range from 4% to 7% or higher. Direct intake of undiluted ACV may irritate the throat, esophagus, or stomach walls. It is critical to dilute ACV correctly before use.

2. Tooth enamel erosion

The acidity of ACV can erode tooth enamel over time, causing dental discomfort and an increased risk of cavities. To prevent this danger, dilute ACV with water or sip with a straw to avoid contact with your teeth. Rinse your mouth with water after taking ACV, and wait at least 30 minutes before brushing your teeth.

3. Gastrointestinal Effects

Some people may feel gastrointestinal discomfort such as bloating, gas, or diarrhea after drinking ACV, especially in large doses or on an empty stomach. Begin with modest doses and evaluate your body's response.

4. Interaction with medications

ACV may interact with some drugs, such as diuretics, insulin, and digoxin. It may drop potassium levels or impact blood sugar levels. If you are taking any drugs, ask your doctor before using ACV on a regular basis.

5. Skin Sensitivity

Undiluted ACV can be harsh on the skin, causing irritation and burns. When using ACV topically, always dilute it and conduct a patch test on a small area of skin before applying it more widely.

- Practical Tips for Safe Use of ACV

To properly incorporate ACV into your daily routine and maximise its advantages, consider the following practical tips:

1. Dilution and Consumption

ACV Tonic: Combine 1-2 tablespoons of ACV and 8-10 ounces of water. If desired, flavor the mixture with honey or a touch of lemon. Begin with a low concentration of ACV and increase gradually as tolerated.

Salad Dressings and Recipes: Add apple cider vinegar to salad dressings, marinades, sauces, and recipes. This not only dilutes the ACV, but also improves its flavor and nutritional benefits.

2. Frequency and dose

Moderation is key: Avoid consuming too much ACV. Most persons can safely consume 1-2 tablespoons diluted in water on a daily basis.

Consume ACV before meals to assist digestion, manage blood sugar levels, and increase fullness. Avoid taking excessive doses of ACV on an empty stomach.

3. Protecting Dental Health.

Drink diluted ACV with a straw to avoid direct contact with tooth enamel.

Rinse and Wait: After ingesting ACV, rinse your mouth with water to neutralize the acidity. Wait at least 30 minutes before cleaning your teeth to avoid enamel deterioration.

4. Skin Applications
When using ACV topically for skincare or haircare, dilute it with water or combine it with other substances to lessen acidity and skin irritation.

Patch Test: To verify your skin tolerates ACV, perform a patch test on a small area of skin before using it more widely.

- Evidence-based Insights and Recommendations
While anecdotal evidence and some studies suggest that ACV may have health benefits, such as improving digestion and blood sugar control, further research is needed to completely understand its effects and optimal use. Here are some evidence-based findings:

Digestive Health: ACV may promote digestion and relieve symptoms such as bloating and indigestion. Its acidic composition can stimulate stomach acid production, which aids in the breakdown of meals.

Blood Sugar Regulation: ACV has been proven in several studies to enhance insulin sensitivity and lower blood sugar levels after meals, which can be advantageous for people who have diabetes or insulin resistance.

Weight Management: According to some research, ACV may help lower hunger and increase feelings of fullness, perhaps aiding weight loss attempts when accompanied with a healthy diet and lifestyle.

- Recipes and Applications With Safety in Mind

Discover these safe and pleasurable ways to add ACV into your diet and everyday routine:

1. ACV Honey Lemonade
Ingredients:

- 1 tablespoon of raw, unfiltered ACV
- Juice from 1/2 lemon
- 1 teaspoon honey.
- 8 ounces of cold water.

Instructions:

- In a glass, mix the ACV, lemon juice, and honey.
- Stir until the honey is dissolved.
- Add the cold water and stir thoroughly.
- Drink this delightful ACV honey lemonade to stay hydrated.

2. ACV-infused salad dressing
Ingredients:

- 1/4 cup of raw, unfiltered ACV
- 1/4 cup extra virgin olive oil.
- 1 tablespoon Dijon mustard.
- 1 teaspoon honey.

- Add salt and pepper to taste.

Instructions:

- In a small mixing bowl, blend ACV, olive oil, Dijon mustard, honey, salt, and pepper until well incorporated.
- Drizzle over salads or marinate meats and veggies.
- Enjoy this delicious ACV-infused dressing to complement your meal.

- Integrating ACV into Various Dietary Preferences

ACV can be tailored to meet a variety of dietary tastes and demands.

Vegan and vegetarian diets: Use apple cider vinegar in dressings, marinades, and beverages to add flavor and potential health advantages without using animal products.

Paleo and Keto Diets: ACV is naturally low in carbs and can be consumed in moderation to supplement these eating patterns.

ACV is naturally gluten-free and dairy-free, making it acceptable for anyone who follow these dietary requirements.

- Tips for Choosing and Storing ACV

To assure the safety and effectiveness of ACV, consider the following tips:

Quality: Select raw, unfiltered ACV with the "mother," a hazy substance that forms naturally during fermentation and is high in healthy enzymes and probiotics.

Organic Options: Choose organic ACV to reduce your exposure to pesticides and other toxins.

To retain ACV's quality and efficacy, store it in a cool, dark place away from direct sunlight.

Incorporating ACV into your daily routine can provide numerous health benefits, but it is critical to utilize it cautiously and responsibly. By following these safety precautions, knowing potential dangers, and incorporating ACV into a healthy food and skincare routine, you may maximize its potential advantages while limiting any potential drawbacks. If you have any specific health issues or conditions, consult your doctor before incorporating ACV into your daily routine. Accept the variety and natural goodness of apple cider vinegar to improve your well-being, with each use a step toward a healthier and more vibrant you.

Chapter 12

FAQs about using apple cider vinegar (ACV) safely and effectively

Here are some commonly asked questions (FAQs) and their responses to help you understand how to use apple cider vinegar (ACV) safely and effectively:

1. Is it safe to eat ACV every day?
Yes, ACV is generally safe for most people to consume in moderation. Begin with tiny doses (1-2 tablespoons diluted in water) and track your body's response. If you are experiencing discomfort, lower the amount or frequency of ingestion.

2. How do I dilute ACV for consumption?
Dilute ACV by combining 1-2 tbsp with 8-10 ounces of water or another beverage. For added taste, try adding honey or a touch of lemon. Consuming undiluted ACV might be harmful to the esophagus and stomach lining.

3. Can ACV help you lose weight?
There is some evidence that ACV may help with weight loss by increasing feelings of fullness, boosting metabolism, and improving insulin sensitivity. However, it is not a cure-all and should be used in conjunction with a well-balanced diet and active lifestyle.

4. Are there any adverse effects from taking ACV?

ACV's potential negative effects include teeth enamel erosion, gastrointestinal discomfort (such as bloating or diarrhea), and skin irritation when applied topically. To reduce hazards, always dilute ACV, safeguard your dental health, and conduct a patch test before applying it to significant regions of skin.

5. Does ACV interfere with medications?

Yes, ACV can interact with some drugs, such as diuretics, insulin, and digoxin. It might impact potassium and blood sugar levels, so if you are taking any medications, talk to your doctor before introducing ACV into your daily routine.

6. How may ACV be used in cooking and recipes?

ACV imparts sour flavor and acidity to salads, marinades, sauces, and beverages. It can also be used in homemade dressings, pickling agents, and beverages such as detox drinks or lemonades. Be imaginative, but keep in mind that it is acidic.

7. Is there a distinction between raw, unfiltered, and ordinary ACV?

Yes, raw, unfiltered ACV contains the "mother," a hazy substance made up of helpful enzymes, proteins, and bacteria produced during fermentation. This gives it more potential health advantages than processed, filtered ACV.

8. How should ACV be stored?

To retain the freshness and potency of ACV, store it in a cool, dark place away from direct sunlight. To avoid contamination, always keep the bottle well packed after each use.

9. Can ACV be used for skin care?

ACV can be used topically to cure acne, soothe sunburn, and balance skin pH. To minimize irritation, always dilute ACV and do a patch test before applying it to wider regions of skin.

10. Should I visit a doctor before using ACV?

If you have any underlying health concerns, are pregnant or nursing, or are using medications, you should contact your doctor before adding ACV to your regular routine. They can offer individualized advise based on your specific health state.

When used properly, apple cider vinegar (ACV) can provide a variety of health benefits. Following these FAQs and suggestions can help you optimize the potential advantages of ACV while reducing any dangers or negative effects. Experiment with ACV in moderation and monitor your body's reaction to identify the optimal method for your health and wellbeing goals.

www.ingramcontent.com/pod-product-compliance
Lightning Source LLC
Chambersburg PA
CBHW050819250726

48653CB00006B/2314